Christoph Eckharter

Nogo in the peripheral nervous system

AF168129

Christoph Eckharter

Nogo in the peripheral nervous system

Natural Sciences Series

Impressum / Imprint

Bibliografische Information der Deutschen Nationalbibliothek: Die Deutsche Nationalbibliothek verzeichnet diese Publikation in der Deutschen Nationalbibliografie; detaillierte bibliografische Daten sind im Internet über http://dnb.d-nb.de abrufbar.
Alle in diesem Buch genannten Marken und Produktnamen unterliegen warenzeichen-, marken- oder patentrechtlichem Schutz bzw. sind Warenzeichen oder eingetragene Warenzeichen der jeweiligen Inhaber. Die Wiedergabe von Marken, Produktnamen, Gebrauchsnamen, Handelsnamen, Warenbezeichnungen u.s.w. in diesem Werk berechtigt auch ohne besondere Kennzeichnung nicht zu der Annahme, dass solche Namen im Sinne der Warenzeichen- und Markenschutzgesetzgebung als frei zu betrachten wären und daher von jedermann benutzt werden dürften.

Bibliographic information published by the Deutsche Nationalbibliothek: The Deutsche Nationalbibliothek lists this publication in the Deutsche Nationalbibliografie; detailed bibliographic data are available in the Internet at http://dnb.d-nb.de.
Any brand names and product names mentioned in this book are subject to trademark, brand or patent protection and are trademarks or registered trademarks of their respective holders. The use of brand names, product names, common names, trade names, product descriptions etc. even without a particular marking in this work is in no way to be construed to mean that such names may be regarded as unrestricted in respect of trademark and brand protection legislation and could thus be used by anyone.

Coverbild / Cover image: www.ingimage.com

Verlag / Publisher:
AV Akademikerverlag
ist ein Imprint der / is a trademark of
OmniScriptum GmbH & Co. KG
Heinrich-Böcking-Str. 6-8, 66121 Saarbrücken, Deutschland / Germany
Email: info@akademikerverlag.de

Herstellung: siehe letzte Seite /
Printed at: see last page
ISBN: 978-3-639-87509-6

Acknowledgment

First of all, I thank Ass.-Prof. Dr. Rüdiger Schweigreiter for the supervision of this diploma thesis. I am especially thankful for the great relationship we had and for giving me space to develop independently and guidance when I encountered problems.

I would also like to thank Univ.-Prof. Dr. Christine Bandtlow for giving me the opportunity to carry out my diploma thesis at the Division of Neurobiochemistry.

Contents

List of Figures

List of Tables

List of abbreviations

a.d. distilled water

bp base pairs

BSA Bovine Serum Albumin

CA cytosine arabinoside

cDNA complementary DNA

CNS central nervous system

div day(s) in vitro

DMEM Dulbecco's Modified Eagle Medium

DPBS Dulbecco's Phosphate-Buffered Saline

DRG dorsal root ganglia

DRGN dorsal root ganglia neurons

EDTA Ethylenediaminetetraacetic acid

ERK extracellular signal-regulated kinase

FBS Fetal Bovine Serum

GFP green fluorescent protein

Fiji (Fiji Is Just) ImageJ

HBSS Hanks' Balanced Salt solution

KO knock-out

L-Gln L-glutamine

LB longest branch

NSF Neural Survival Factor

TAE Tris-acetate-EDTA

TBST Tris-Buffered Saline with Tween 20

TNIS total number of intersections

TNL total neurite length

o/n overnight

p postnatal

PBS Phosphate-Buffered Saline

PCR polymerase chain reaction

PNS peripheral nervous system

PFA paraformaldehyde

PI3K phosphatidylinositol-3 kinase

PLL Poly-L-lysine

PNBM Primary Neuron Basal Medium

RHD reticulon homology domain

rpm revolutions per minute

RT room temperature

RTKs receptor tyrosine kinases

rxn reaction

SC Schwann cell

SDS sodium dodecyl sulfate

SEM standard error of the mean

siRNA small interfering RNA

v/v volume per volume

WT wild-type

1 Abstract

While a lot of research effort in the last decade was devoted to understand the role of Nogo-A in the central nervous system (CNS), not much is currently known about another Nogo isoform, namely Nogo-B. Recent experiments in our laboratory revealed that Nogo-B is enriched in Schwann cells of the peripheral nervous system (PNS) and could play an important role in axonal branching of sensory neurons.

In this diploma thesis, we established co-cultures of Schwann cells and dorsal root ganglia (DRG) sensory neurons to assess the role of Nogo in the PNS. With the use of Nogo knock-out (KO) mice, we found that Nogo is a promotor of axonal branching. The total neurite length (TNL) and the total number of axonal branch points of dorsal root ganglia neurons (DRGN) cultured on Nogo KO Schwann cells were significantly decreased compared to DRGN that were grown on wild-type (WT) Schwann cells. Importantly, we did not see any difference of the longest branch (LB), which means that elongative axon growth is not affected by Nogo.

Further, we tried to investigate whether the observed branch-promoting effect is mediated through a direct, physical interaction between Schwann cells and neurons or via an indirect, non-physical interaction through molecules secreted by Schwann cells. Preliminary experiments suggest that Schwann cell expressed Nogo influences neuronal morphology also in an indirect, non-physical manner. Future experiments with a refined technical approach will provide a definitive answer to the question of an indirect interference.

Taken together, this diploma thesis revealed that Schwann cell expressed Nogo promotes axonal branching of sensory neurons and that this effect seems to be mediated primarily by a direct cell surface interaction between Schwann cells and neurons.

2 Zusammenfassung

Im letzten Jahrzehnt beschäftigten sich viele Forschungsgruppen damit, die Funktion von Nogo-A im zentralen Nervensystem (ZNS) zu verstehen. Eine zweite Isoform des Nogo-Gens, Nogo-B, blieb weitestgehend unerforscht. Kürzlich durchgeführte Experimente unseres Labors zeigten, dass Nogo-B in Schwannzellen des peripheren Nervensystems (PNS) exprimiert wird und an der Bildung axonaler Verzweigungen von sensorischen Nervenzellen beteiligt sein könnte.

Im Zuge dieser Diplomarbeit kultivierten wir Schwannzellen mit aus Spinalganglien isolierten sensorischen Nervenzellen, um mehr über Nogo's Funktion im PNS herauszufinden. Die Experimente wurden mit Nogo knock-out (KO) Mäusen durchgeführt und zeigten, dass Nogo die Bildung axonaler Verzweigungen fördert. Die Gesamtneuritenlänge und die Gesamtanzahl an axonalen Verzweigungspunkten waren signifikant erhöht, wenn die sensorischen Nervenzellen mit Nogo KO Schwannzellen, im Vergleich zu wild-typ (WT) Schwannzellen, kultiviert wurden. Weiters konnten wir keinen Unterschied im Längenwachstum der Neuriten beobachten, woraus wir ableiten, dass Nogo das Längenwachstum der Neuriten nicht beeinflusst.

Nachdem wir beweisen konnten, dass Nogo an der Bildung von axonalen Verzweigungspunkten beteiligt ist, wollten wir herausfinden, ob dieser Effekt über eine direkte, physische Interaktion zwischen Schwannzellen und Nervenzellen, oder über einen indirekten, nicht-physischen Mechanismus durch Moleküle, die von Schwannzellen sezerniert werden, vermittelt wird. In vorläufigen Experimenten konnten wir nachweisen, dass Nogo die Nervenzellmorphologie auch über einen indirekten Mechanismus beeinflusst. Für eine definitive Antwort benötigen wir jedoch noch zusätzliche Experimente, die wir mit einem leicht modifizierten experimentellen Ansatz durchführen werden.

Zusammenfassend fanden wir durch diese Diplomarbeit heraus, dass Nogo an der Bildung axonaler Verzweigungen von sensorischen Nervenzellen beteiligt ist und dieser Effekt hauptsächlich durch eine direkte Zelloberflächeninteraktion zwischen Schwannzellen und Nervenzellen vermittelt wird.

3 Personal contribution

After an introduction into laboratory work and the experimental procedure by the supervisor, the author of the diploma thesis conducted most experiments on his own.

The author was in close contact with the supervisor and results or problems were discussed intensely. When the author was not able to perform experimental work due to classes at university or private appointments, the supervisor filled in for him (e.g. fixation of co-cultures or mating of mice).

In total, nineteen experiments were conducted for this diploma thesis. Sixteen experiments were done by the author, two by the supervisor and one by Nina Juncker, another thesis student.

4 Introduction

Whereas nerve fibers in the lesioned CNS can not regenerate, regenerative growth of nerve fibers after injury takes place in the PNS. However, regeneration in the PNS carries a few problems (Figure 4.1). Misdirected axonal growth with regenerating axons not reinnervating the original targets or axonal sprouting, which leads to innervation of more than one target by the regenerating axon, are just two mechanisms that cause troubles for patients.

An example of axonal sprouting is the reinnervation of antagonizing muscle groups by a single regenerating motoneuron, which can be the cause of abnormally associated movements [1]. Other troubles like disturbed sensory localization or fine motor control, or even maladaptive changes, such as neuropathic pain, hyperreflexia and dystonia may also result from peripheral nerve injuries [2].

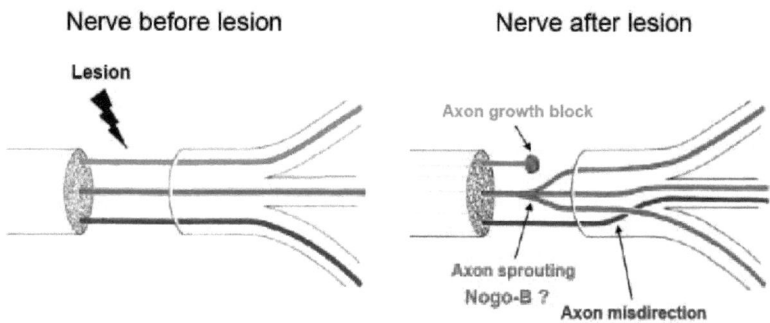

Figure 4.1: Problems of regenerating peripheral nerve fibers (Schematic adapted from [1])

An important role for axonal regrowth plays remyelination of the regenerating axons by Schwann cells [3] and the communication between these two cell types, which is either directly via cell surface proteins or indirectly by secreted neurotrophic factors and neuropoietic cytokines [4], [5].
Schwann cells thus create an environment that is highly supportive for axonal growth. The problem is that many involved molecules are also stimulators of axonal branching and hence promote the occurrence of the above mentioned nerve regeneration problems [1].

One potentially interesting protein in the communication between Schwann cells and neurons is Nogo-B, which is a protein isoform of the RTN4/Nogo gene. Via alternative splicing and differential promotor usage, the three main isoforms Nogo-A/B/C are derived from the Nogo gene [6]. Not only the structural features are different (Figure 4.2), the protein isoforms are also specified by their expression pattern.
While Nogo-A is primarily expressed in oligodendroctyes and neurons of the CNS [7], Nogo-B is enriched in endothelial and smooth muscle cells of blood vessels [8] and in Schwann cells of the PNS [Schweigreiter R, unpublished].

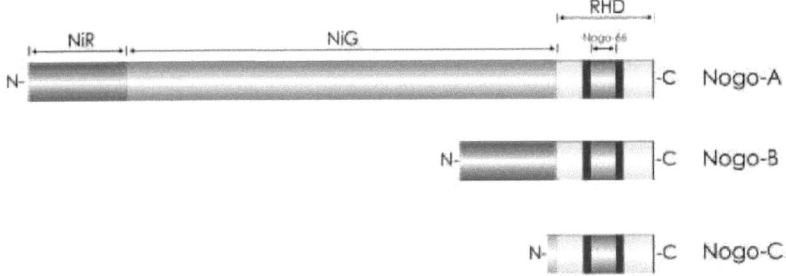

Figure 4.2: Three different Nogo isoforms. The C-terminal RHD is shared by all three isoforms (Schematic adapted from Schweigreiter R).

Down-regulation experiments with Nogo-B in Schwann cells using small interfering RNA (siRNA) had indicated that Schwann cell expressed Nogo-B influences the morphology of co-cultured sensory neurons derived from DRG [Schweigreiter R, unpublished].

The knock-down of Nogo-B in Schwann cells with siRNA, however, was not efficient, it reduced Nogo-B by not more than 50%. To solve this problem, we intended to perform the co-culture experiments with Nogo KO mice that are completely devoid of Nogo-A and Nogo-B [9].

5 Aims of the thesis

The first aim of the thesis was to carry out the Schwann cell/DRGN co-culture experiments with wild-type (Nogo +/+) and Nogo deficient (Nogo -/-) Schwann cells and analyze the morphology of co-cultured DRGN.

The second aim of the thesis was to find out if the branching effect on neuronal morphology, that we have found and characterized in the first part of the thesis, is mediated through a direct, physical interaction between neurons and Schwann cells or via an indirect interaction mediated by molecules secreted from Schwann cells.

6 Material and methods

6.1 Mice

Postnatal day 3-4 C57BL6/N male and female WT, Nogo-A/B KO and heterozygous Nogo-A/B KO mice were used for the isolation of Schwann cells.

DRGN were isolated from adult (between 2 and 3 months old) C57BL6/J and C57BL6/N male and female mice.

6.1.1 Breeding scheme of heterozygous Nogo-A/B KO mice

Heterozygous Nogo-A/B KO mice were used for breeding to obtain Nogo-A/B KO, heterozygous Nogo-A/B KO and WT littermates used in the experiments.

Two females were paired with one male together for 2 days, before the male was removed from the cage. If a mouse looked pregnant after about 15 days, the two females were separated.
Female mice were 6 to 8 weeks old and male mice were some weeks older when they were first used for breeding.
After giving birth, tail biopsies from one or two day old pups were taken (Section 6.2.1) and littermates were either used for experiments or left with their mother until weaning, 4 weeks after birth.

6.2 Molecular biology

6.2.1 Isolation of genomic DNA from mouse tails

Tail biopsies of about two millimeters in length were taken from one or two day old pups. A biopsy was then transferred into a 2 ml Eppendorf tube filled with 0.5 ml of lysis buffer (Table 6.1) and rotated at 55°C in a hybridization oven for a minimum of four hours. Following complete lysis, the Eppendorf tube was spun in a centrifuge for 5 minutes at 14000 revolutions per minute (rpm). The supernatant was poured into a 1.5 ml Eppendorf tube filled with 0.5 ml of isopropanol. The tube was gently shaken until precipitation of DNA was complete. The DNA was then transferred with tweezers into a 2 ml Eppendorf tube filled with 80 µl of Buffer TE and rotated at 55°C for a minimum of eight hours.

Table 6.1: Lysis buffer

Substance	Concentration
Tris pH 8.5	100 mM
EDTA	5 mM
SDS	0.2%
NaCl	200 mM
Proteinase K	100 µg/ml

Proteinase K was always added fresh.

6.2.2 Polymerase chain reaction

A master mix was made and 23 µl aliquots were put into 0.2 ml thin-walled tubes. Two µl of each dissolved DNA sample (Section 6.2.1) was added into a tube, making it up to a total volume of 25 µl (Table 6.2). A cooling block was used during the pipetting process to prevent the polymerase chain reaction (PCR) from starting. Finally, amplification (Table 6.3) of DNA was performed in a thermal cycler.

Because the primers for the detection of the WT and the Nogo KO allele could not be used together, two different master mixes were prepared. For the detection of the WT allele, the master mix contained the forward primer nogoWT_1s and the reverse primer nogoWT_1as, whereas the master mix for the detection of the Nogo KO allele contained the same forward primer nogoWT_1s, but the reverse primer IRES200R (Table 6.4).

The size of the amplicon of the WT-reaction (rxn) was 385 base pairs (bp). The amplicon of the KO-rxn was about 100 bp larger.

Table 6.2: PCR reaction mix

Substance	Volume
10x Pfu Buffer with $MgSO_4$	2.5 µl
$MgSO_4$ [25 mM]	1.5 µl
Forward Primer [10 µM]	0.5 µl
Reverse Primer [10 µM]	0.5 µl
dNTP [25 µM]	0.2 µl
Taq Polymerase	0.3 µl
DNA	2 µl
a.d.	17.5 µl
	total 25 µl

Table 6.3: PCR amplification program

Step	Time	Temperature
1. Initial denaturation	3 min	95°C
2. Denaturation	30 sec	95°C
3. Annealing	30 sec	65°C
4. Extension	45 sec	72°C
5. Final extension	5 min	72°C
6. Cooling	endless	4°C

The amplification procedure (steps 2-4) was repeated 39 times.

Table 6.4: Primer sequences

Name	Primer sequence
nogoWT_1s	5'-TGT GGC CTT TGC GGG TTC CTC-3'
nogoWT_1as	5'-ACC GAG TCG CTG CTG AAG TCC-3'
IRES200R	5'-AGA GGA ACT GCT TCC TTC AC-3'

6.2.3 Agarose gel electrophoresis

DNA fragments were separated by horizontal gel electrophoresis using an agarose gel. Gels were made by heating 2% agarose in 1x Tris-acetate-EDTA (TAE) buffer (Table 6.5) and adding Ethidium bromide (5 µl per 100 ml gel solution) to the solution. After the gel had hardened, it was covered with 1x TAE buffer.

Two point eight µl of 10x loading dye was added to the tube with the amplified PCR product (Section 6.2.2) before the sample was pipetted into the gel pockets. Between 3 to 5 µl of Ethidium bromide was pipetted to the top and the bottom of the gel chamber and the gel was run at a constant voltage (10 V/cm gel length). Final documentation of the gel was made with an UV-light imaging system.

Table 6.5: 1x TAE buffer

Substance	Concentration
Tris base	40 mM
Acetic acid	20 mM
EDTA	1 mM
dissolved in a.d.	

6.3 Cell culture

6.3.1 Solutions for cell cultures

Table 6.6: Supplemented DMEM

Basal Medium	Supplement	Concentration
DMEM supplemented with	FBS	10% (v/v)
	L-Gln	1% (v/v)
	Penicillin/Streptomycin	1% (v/v)

Table 6.7: PNBM medium

Basal Medium	Supplement	Concentration
PNBM supplemented with	NSF-1	1:50 (v/v)
	L-Gln	1:100 (v/v)
	Gentamycin/Amphotericin B	1:1000 (v/v)

Table 6.8: 10x HBSS

Substance	Concentration
KCl	53.64 mM
$Na_2HPO_4 * 2H_2O$	5.05 mM
KH_2PO_4	4.4 mM
$NaHCO_3$	41.66 mM
NaCl	1.37 mM
D-Glucose	55.5 mM

dissolved in a.d.; pH 7.4; working conc. 1x

Table 6.9: 10x PBS-EDTA

Substance	Concentration
NaCl	1.368 M
KCl	26.8 mM
$Na_2HPO_4 * 2H_2O$	100 mM
KH_2PO_4	20 mM
EDTA	6.72 mM

dissolved in a.d.; pH 7.4; working conc. 1x

BSA medium (3.5%)

First, 1.75 g of Bovine Serum Albumin (BSA) was put into a 50 ml tube. Then the tube was filled up to 45 ml with Dulbecco's Modified Eagle Medium (DMEM) and the BSA was dissolved on a horizontal shaker. After complete dissolution, the solution was sterile filtered using a 0.2 micron filter. Finally, the tube was filled up to 50 ml with DMEM.

Trypsin (0.05%)

A 20 ml solution of 0.05% Trypsin was made with 0.4 ml Trypsin 2.5%, 19.6 ml 1x HBSS (Table 6.8) and 14.71 μl 10x PBS-EDTA (Table 6.9). Subsequently working aliquots of 2 ml were made and stored at -20°C.

6.3.2 Isolation and culture of Schwann cells

Schwann cells were isolated from the sciatic nerves of a 3 or 4 day old mouse. Both sciatic nerves were dissected and collected into Dulbecco's Phosphate-Buffered Saline (DPBS) on ice. Afterwards the nerves were transferred with tweezers into 12 ml tubes containing 500 µl of DPBS.

Zero point five ml of a 5 mg/ml solution of collagenase type I (collagenase was freshly dissolved in DPBS) was added and the nerves were incubated at 37°C for 7 min. The next step was to remove 100 µl volume, replace with 100 µl of a solution of 2.5% Trypsin and incubate at 37°C for 5 min. During these two steps of incubation, the nerves were swirled from time to time.

Enzyme digestion was stopped by adding 2 ml of supplemented DMEM (Table 6.6). Three µl of DNase I (working concentration was 0.01 mg/ml) were added and the nerves were triturated with a fire-polished Pasteur pipette with 15 gentle strokes. After sedimentation of tissue fragments, approximately two-thirds of the supernatant was decanted into a 15 ml tube. Another round of trituration with 15 harsher strokes was started after adding 2 ml of supplemented DMEM and 2 µl of DNase I. This round's supernatant was pooled with that of the first round.

The cell suspension was centrifuged with 290 g for 10 min at room temperature (RT). The supernatant was discarded and the pellet was resuspended with the fire-polished Pasteur pipette in 1 ml of supplemented DMEM.

The isolated Schwann cells were counted with a Neubauer chamber and plated onto a Poly-L-lysine (PLL) coated coverslip at a density of $1.2 \cdot 10^5$ cells/cm^2. The coverslip was located in a well of a 48-microwell plate and coating was for at least 2 hours at 37°C and 5% CO_2. Finally, the cells were placed in the incubator at 37°C and 8.5% CO_2 in humidified air overnight (o/n).

Regardless which experimental set-up (direct or indirect; difference between set-ups is explained in Section 6.3.3) was used, several hours before the DRGN were added to the Schwann cell culture, the medium in the well was changed from supplemented DMEM to Primary Neuron Basal Medium (PNBM) medium supplemented with 2 µM cytosine arabinoside (CA). After changing the medium, the Schwann cell culture was stored again in the incubator at 37°C and 5% CO_2 in humidified air until the neurons were added.

6.3.3 Isolation of DRGN and co-culture with Schwann cells

Neurons were isolated from the DRG of an adult (between two and three months old) mouse.
The spine was dissected and cut into two or three pieces. After splitting the pieces longitudinally, they were placed into DPBS on ice. Then piece after piece was taken and the DRG of the thoraco-lumbal region were pulled out. The nerve trunks were cut off and the DRG were put into DPBS on ice. After a minimum of twelve DRG were collected, they were transferred into a 15 ml tube using a low retention tip with a large opening.

After washing the DRG with Phosphate-Buffered Saline (PBS), 0.5 ml of Liberase DL was added and the DRG were incubated at 37°C for 35 min. The Liberase (stock was 2.5 mg/ml) was diluted 1:10 (v/v) with DMEM. After this incubation step, the Liberase was replaced with another 0.5 ml of it and incubated again at 37°C for 35 min. Subsequently, the DRG were washed twice with PBS, 2 ml of 0.05% Trypsin (Section 6.3.1) was added and incubated at 37°C for 30 min. During the incubation steps, the DRG were swirled from time to time to prevent them from sticking together at the bottom of the tube.

Following the trypsin incubation, the DRG were washed twice with PBS before 0.75 ml of PNBM medium (Table 6.7) were added. The medium was stored at 37°C for approximately 1 hour before it was used.

The DRG were triturated with a fire-polished Pasteur pipette with 15 gentle strokes. After sedimentation of debris, the supernatant was decanted into a 15 ml tube. Another round of trituration with 15 harsher strokes was started after adding another 0.75 ml of PNBM medium. The second round's supernatant was pooled with that of the first round.

Seven point five ml of 3.5% BSA medium (Section 6.3.1) were put into a 15 ml tube and the DRGN suspension was gently added on top using the fire-polished Pasteur pipette. The tube was exactly counterbalanced and centrifuged with 14 g for 15 min at RT. After centrifugation, most of the supernatant was discarded and the pellet was resuspended with the fire-polished Pasteur pipette in a total of 250 µl of PNBM medium.

6.3.3.1 Direct co-culture

After resuspension of pellet, the isolated DRGN were counted with a Neubauer chamber and plated directly onto the Schwann cell culture that had been prepared the day before (Figure 6.1). The neurons were plated at a density of 1200 cells/cm^2.

Finally, the Schwann cell (SC)/DRGN co-culture was placed in the incubator at 37°C and 5% CO_2 in humidified air for 13.5 to 14 hours until fixation.

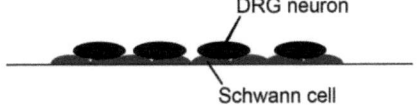

Figure 6.1: Schematic front view of a direct co-culture. Schwann cells are shown in blue, DRGN in black.

6.3.3.2 Indirect co-culture

In contrast to the direct co-culture, the isolated DRGN were plated onto a separate PLL/Laminin coated coverslip at a density of 1900 to 2000 cells/cm^2 and stored in the incubator at 37°C and 5% CO_2 for about 1 hour and 45 minutes pre-incubation time.

The coverslip was located in a well of a 48-microwell plate and coating was first with PLL at 37°C and 5% CO_2 for at least 2 hours. After washing the coverslip three times with Hanks' Balanced Salt solution (HBSS) (Table 6.8), it was coated with Laminin at 37°C and 5% CO_2 for at least 2 hours. Laminin was dissolved in HBSS at a concentration of 10 µg/ml. The coverslip was washed twice with HBSS and the neurons were plated onto it immediately.

After pre-incubation, the coverslip with the DRGN was taken out of the well with tweezers and put face-down onto the Schwann cell culture from the previous day. Because the coverslip was prepared in a special way (little droplets of paraffin, so-called paraffin feet, were added to the edge, as shown in Figure 6.2a), there was no direct cell surface contact between neurons and Schwann cells (Figure 6.2b).

Finally, the SC/DRGN co-culture was placed again in the incubator at 37°C and 5% CO_2 in humidified air for 13.5 hours until fixation.

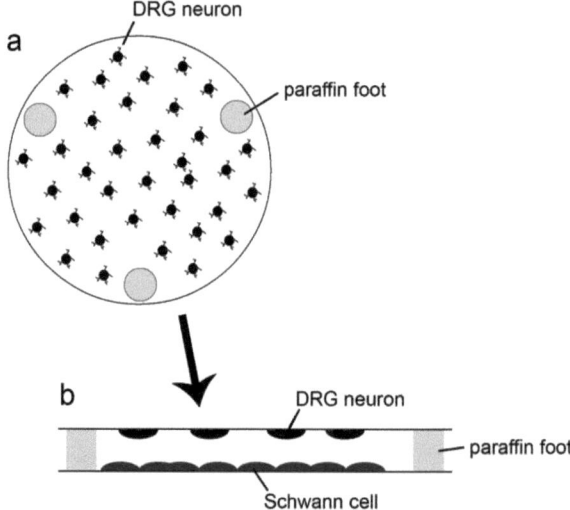

Figure 6.2: Two schematic views of an indirect co-culture. (**a**) Bottom view of the PLL/Laminin coated coverslip with DRGN. (**b**) Front view of an indirect co-culture. Schwann cells are shown in blue, DRGN in black.

6.4 Immunocytochemistry

6.4.1 Solutions for immunocytochemistry

Table 6.10: Blocking solution

Substance	Concentration
Goat Serum	3% (v/v)
BSA	1%
Triton X-100	0.1% (v/v)
dissolved in PBS; sterile filtered	

Table 6.11: TBST

Substance	Concentration
Tris base	50 mM
NaCl	150 mM
Tween 20	0.1% (v/v)
dissolved in a.d.; sterile filtered	

PFA solution (4%)

To obtain a solution of 4% paraformaldehyde (PFA), the PFA was dissolved in an appropriate amount of PBS at 70°C with regular shaking for no longer than 30 min. After complete dissolution, the solution was supplemented with 5% Sucrose.

6.4.2 Fixation

Co-cultures were fixed in two steps in order to prevent disruption of fragile DRGN cell bodies. First, in a pre-fixation step, medium volume was reduced to 0.5 ml per well and 0.5 ml of PFA solution was added for 10 min at RT. In the second fixation step all liquid was removed and 0.5 ml of the PFA solution was added for another 10 min at RT. Finally, the coverslips were washed three times with PBS and either used immediately for immunostaining (see Section 6.4.3) or the 48-microwell plate was sealed with Parafilm and stored at 4°C for later use.

6.4.3 Immunostaining

To avoid unspecific binding, the co-culture was first incubated with a minimum volume of 250 µl blocking solution (Table 6.10) per well for at least 1 hour at RT. Then the primary antibody was added and the co-culture was stored at 4°C o/n. As primary antibody we used either N52 (anti-Neurofilament 200 antibody) at 1:500 dilution or TuJ-1 (anti-beta III Tubulin antibody) at 1:2000 dilution. The antibodies were diluted in blocking solution.

Following the first incubation step, the co-culture was washed three times with Tris-Buffered Saline with Tween 20 (TBST) (Table 6.11) and incubated with the secondary antibody for 2 hours at RT, wrapped in aluminum foil in order to prevent bleaching of the fluorophore. As secondary antibody we used goat anti-mouse IgG conjugated with the fluorophore Alexa Fluor 488 (1:1000 dilution in blocking solution).

The co-culture was washed three times with TBST and afterwards incubated for nuclear staining with Hoechst diluted 1:10000 in distilled water (a.d.) for about a minute at RT. This step was performed to wash away remaining salt crystals. Finally, the coverslip was mounted face-down on an object slide with a droplet of DAKO mounting medium. For a coverslip of the indirect experimental set-up, the paraffin feet were removed prior to mounting. The object slide was stored at 4°C o/n to allow the mounting medium to solidify before starting microscopic analysis.

6.5 Neuron analysis

A Zeiss Axio Imager.M2 microscope was used to obtain images of the fluorescent-labeled neurons. Images were taken at 20x magnification. Image processing was performed with the software (Fiji Is Just) ImageJ (Fiji).

6.5.1 Optimization of images

With Fiji, the color depth of the images was converted from 16-bit to 8-bit Grayscale and neurons that did not fit into one image due to the image area limitation of the CCD camera were assembled together using the "2D Stitching" function (Figure 6.4).

To make skeletonization of neurons (Section 6.5.2) easier, all neurons and structures other than the desired one were removed from the images (Figure 6.3).

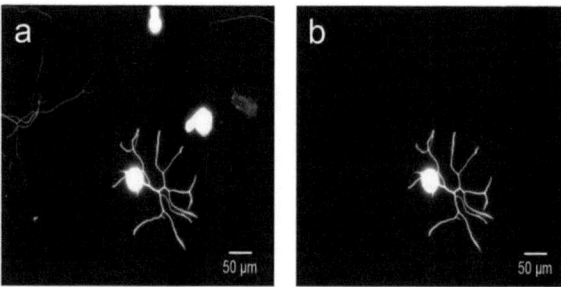

Figure 6.3: Optimization of an image. (**a**) Raw image. (**b**) Optimized image. All irrelevant neurons and structures were removed.

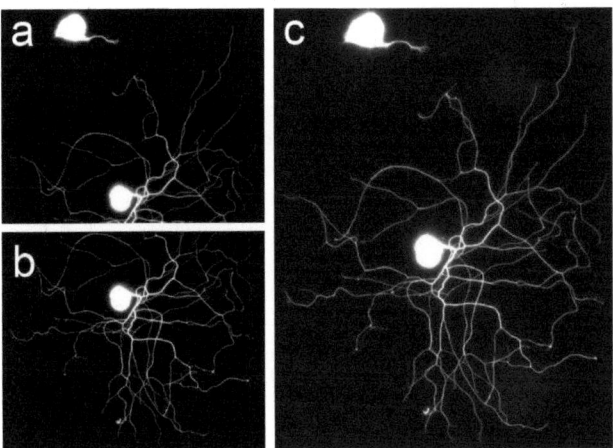

Figure 6.4: Image Stitching with Fiji. (**a**) Image of the upper part of the neuron. (**b**) Image of the lower part of the neuron. (**c**) Final image that was created by stitching together the neuronal parts from Figure a and b.

6.5.2 Skeletonization of neurons

As shown in Figure 6.5, the optimized images were loaded with the WIS-NeuroMath software [10], [11] one after another. Each image was executed with individual parameters to get an ideal skeleton of the neuron (see Figure 6.6a).

The following parameters were individualized:

- *Noise Level*
  With this setting the sensitivity of neurite detection was adjusted. If set too low, the software added artificial neurites, especially when there was a lot of background noise. If set too high, some neurites were not detected.
  Values between 1 and 2 were used most of the time. "Auto Calc Noise" was used for images of indirect co-culture experiments (Section 6.3.3.2) because there was little to no background noise which was due to the culturing of neurons on a glass surface rather than on a Schwann cell layer.

- *Min Cell Intensity*
  A minimum threshold value for the detection of the cell body. Because the color depth of the images was set to 8-bit Grayscale, values between 0 and 255 were possible. If set too low, the detected cell body was too large. If set too high, only a small or no cell body was detected. A value of 200 was used most of the time.

The value of the parameter *Units* depends on the resolution of the microscope objective. Throughout our experiments we used a 20x objective. According to the manufacturer's specifications, 1 pixel equates to 0.37 μm, which means that 1 μm equates to 2.703 pixels.

The parameters *Min Area*, *Max Area* and *Min Diameter* referred to the cell body of the neuron and could be used to exclude neurons other than the desired one. Because undesired neurons were removed from the images (Section 6.5.1), the values of these parameters were set to 200 μm^2, 4000 μm^2 and 20 μm, respectively. Only *Min Diameter* was adjusted to lower values for some neurons.

All other parameters were left at default settings.

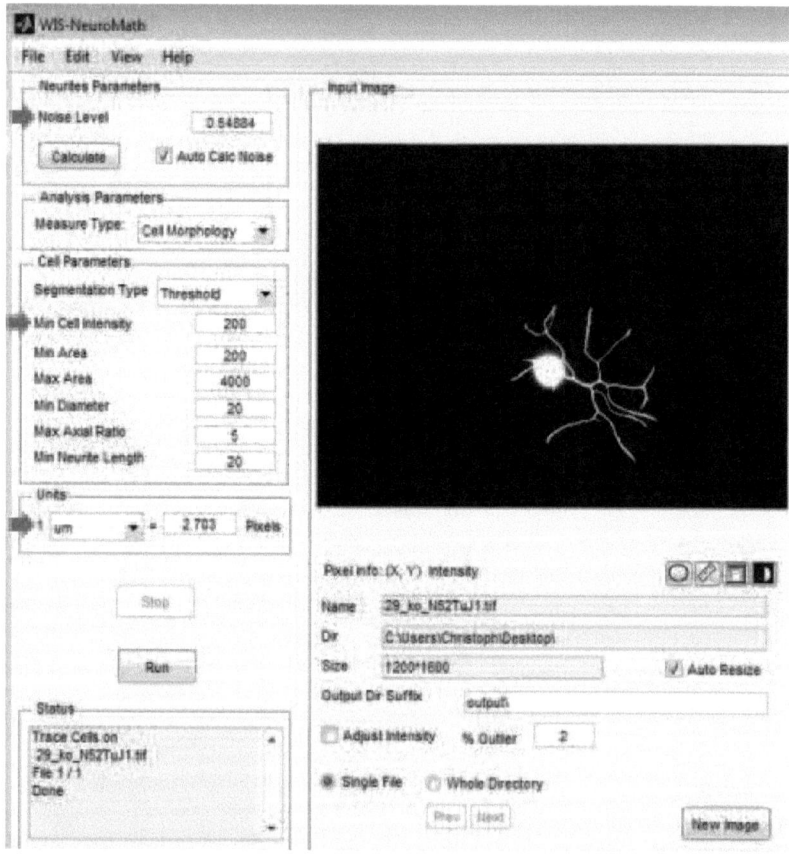

Figure 6.5: Extract of the user interface of WIS-NeuroMath. The red arrows indicate important settings (*Noise Level*, *Min Cell Intensity* and *Units*).

With the skeletonization process bitmap images (.bmp files) of the neurons were generated by the software (Figure 6.6a). Depending on the size of the original images, WIS-NeuroMath reduced the size of the bitmap images to either the half or to one-third of the original size (e.g. from 1600x1200 to 800x600).

The software also generated text files containing morphological characteristics of the skeletonized neurons (e.g. total neurite length and longest branch).

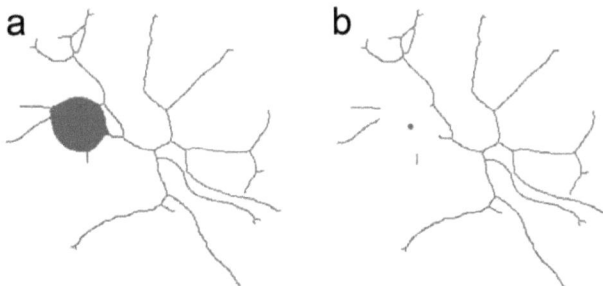

Figure 6.6: Skeletonized neuron. (**a**) Before removal of the cell body. (**b**) After removal of the cell body. A point marks the center of the cell body.

Before Sholl analysis (Section 6.5.3) could be performed, the cell body of all neurons was removed with the Adobe Photoshop CS2 software. The center of the cell body was marked with a point (Figure 6.6b), which was important for the subsequent Sholl analysis.

6.5.3 Sholl analysis

Sholl analysis was carried out using Fiji's "Sholl Analysis" function. The bitmap images of the neuronal skeletons were first subjected to Fiji's "Make Binary" function, resulting in .tif files.

Subsequently, the units of measurement of the "Sholl Analysis" function were set to appropriate values. Because the image size of the skeletonized neurons was reduced, as described in Section 6.5.2, it was necessary to adapt the units of measurement for all neurons.

Depending on the reduction of the original image size, the following units of measurement were used:

- Reduction by half: 1 pixel = 0.74 μm
- Reduction to one-third: 1 pixel = 1.11 μm

Finally, the center of analysis, which was defined as the center of the cell body (Figure 6.6b), was selected with the point selection tool and the "Sholl Analysis" function was executed for each neuron separately using the following parameters:

- *Starting radius*: 0 µm

- *Ending radius*: infinite

- *Radius step size*: 10 µm

Figure 6.7 schematically shows how the "Sholl Analysis" function draws concentric circles around the center of the cell body and measures the number of neurite intersections with each circle. The distance between two circles was 10 µm.

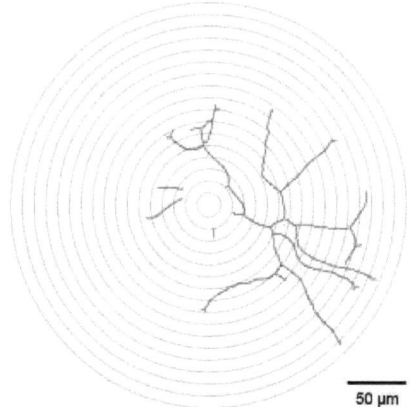

50 µm

Figure 6.7: Schematic of Sholl analysis of a skeletonized neuron

As a result, a spreadsheet file containing the number of neurite intersections for each concentric circle was created for every analyzed neuron.

6.5.4 Diameter of the cell body

The shortest diameter of the cell body was measured with Fiji for every neuron. Because the original images that were taken with the microscope were used as a source, no adaptation of the units of measurement was necessary for individual images.

The following units of measurement were used:

- 1 pixel = 0.37 µm

6.5.5 Consolidation of data

For each experiment a spreadsheet file containing the morphological characteristics of all analyzed neurons was created. The neurons were separated by the genotype and for every neuron the following characteristics were documented:

- Diameter of the cell body

- Total neurite length (TNL)

- Longest branch (LB)

- Number of neurite intersections for each concentric circle

- Total number of neurite intersections (TNIS)
  The number of neurite intersections with all concentric circles drawn around a neuron.

The mean of total neurite length, longest branch and total number of intersections was calculated for each genotype and used for statistical analysis.

6.6 Statistics

Statistical analysis was performed using the software SigmaPlot 12.5 (Systat Software). A two-tailed one-sample t-test was used for analysis and the results were reported as mean $\pm$ SEM for TNL, LB and total number of intersections (TNIS). A p-value of ≤ 0.05 was considered statistically significant.

6.7 Chemicals

Table 6.12: List of used chemicals

Substance	Company	Product No.
1% Ethidium bromide solution	ROTH	2218.1
2-Propanol	ROTH	6752.1
2.5% Trypsin	Gibco	15090
Acetic acid	Sigma-Aldrich	33209
Agarose	Sigma-Aldrich	A9539
Alexa Fluor 488 Goat Anti-Mouse IgG Antibody	Life Technologies	A-11029
Bovine Serum Albumin	Sigma-Aldrich	A7906
Buffer TE	QIAGEN	1018499
Collagenase, Type I	Gibco	17100-017
Cytosine arabinoside	Sigma-Aldrich	C1768
D-Glucose	Sigma	G7021
DMEM High Glucose	PAA	E15-009
DNA Ladder, 1kb	Promega	G5711
DNase I	Roche	11284932001
dNTP	Thermo Scientific	R0181
DPBS	Sigma-Aldrich	D4031
EDTA	ROTH	8043.1
Fetal Bovine Serum	PAA	A15-101
Fluorescence Mounting Medium	Dako	S3023
Goat Serum	PAA	B11-035
Hoechst 33342	Sigma-Aldrich	B2261
KCl	AppliChem	A3582
KH_2PO_4	AppliChem	A3620

Substance	Company	Product No.
L-Glutamin	Sigma-Aldrich	59202C
Laminin	Sigma-Aldrich	L2020
Liberase DL	Roche	05401160001
N52 Monoclonal Antibody	Sigma-Aldrich	N0142
NaCl	ROTH	HN00.3
NaHCO$_3$	AppliChem	A1940
Na$_2$HPO$_4$ $*$ 2H$_2$O	AppliChem	A3905
Orange G	AppliChem	A1404
Paraformaldehyde	ROTH	0335.2
PBS	PAA	H15-002
PCR water	Sigma-Aldrich	95284
Penicillin-Streptomycin	Sigma-Aldrich	P0781
Pfu DNA Polymerase	Fermentas	EP0502
PNGM Primary Neuron Growth Medium BulletKit	Lonza	CC-4461
Poly-L-lysine	Sigma-Aldrich	P4707
Primers	Sigma-Aldrich	
Proteinase K	Promega	V3021
SDS	Sigma-Aldrich	L4509
Sucrose	Sigma-Aldrich	16104
Taq Polymerase	selfmade	
Tris base	Sigma-Aldrich	93352
Triton X-100	Sigma-Aldrich	T9284
Trypsin	Sigma-Aldrich	T4549
TuJ-1 Monoclonal Antibody	R&D Systems	MAB1195
Tween 20	ROTH	9127.1

6.8 Instruments

Table 6.13: List of used instruments

Instrument	Company	Type
Centrifuge	Eppendorf	5810
Centrifuge	Hettich	Mikro 200
CO2 Incubator	Memmert	INC 108
CO2 Incubator	Thermo Electron Corporation	Heraeus HERAcell 150
Fisherbrand Low Retention Tips	Fisher Scientific	02-717-156
Fluorescence Microscope	Zeiss	Axio Imager.M2
Gel Documentation System	peqlab	1100
Hybridization Oven	Biometra	OV1
Objective	Zeiss	Plan-Apochromat 20x/0.8
PCR tubes	STARLAB	I1402-4300
Stereoscopic Zoom Microscope	Nikon	SMZ800
Thermal Cycler	MJ Research	PTC-200

6.9 Software

Table 6.14: List of used software

Software	Provider	Version
Fiji	free software	1.48g
MetaVue Research Imaging Software	Molecular Devices	5.0r2
Office	Microsoft	2007
Photoshop	Adobe	CS2
Prism	GraphPad Software	6.01
SigmaPlot	Systat Software	12.5.0.38
Wis-NeuroMath	Weizmann Institute of Science	3.4.8

7 Results

7.1 Experimental procedure and problems

The following section gives an overview to better understand how data was generated and delineates major problems that occurred. Figure 7.1 illustrates the entire experimental procedure.

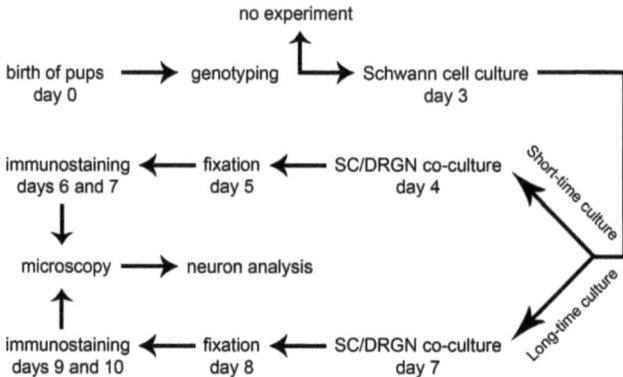

Figure 7.1: Flowchart of entire experimental procedure

7.1.1 Genotyping

After the DNA was extracted from tail biopsies of one or two day old pups (Section 6.2.1), DNA samples were analyzed by PCR (Section 6.2.2) with primers specific for the WT allele and the Nogo KO allele (Table 6.4).

Figure 7.2 shows a typical gel electrophoresis result (Section 6.2.3) of DNA samples of a litter of eight mice. A band in the upper part represents a positive Nogo KO allele, while a band in the bottom part represents a positive WT allele.

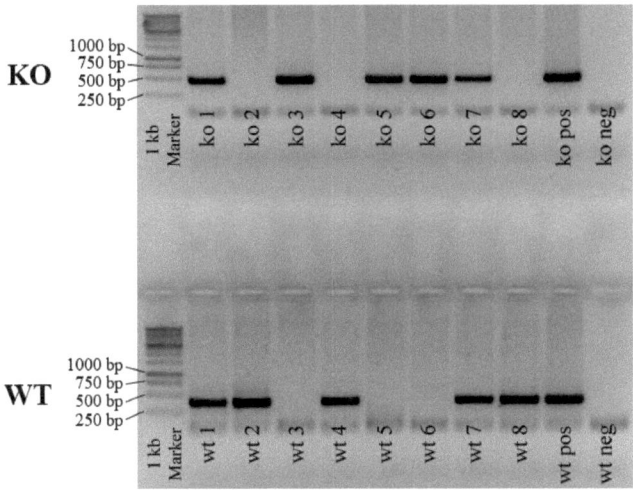

Figure 7.2: Gel electrophoresis of eight DNA samples from mouse tails. Nogo KO alleles are revealed in the upper part, while the lower part shows WT alleles. A band indicates a positive allele. A heterozygous Nogo KO mouse sample (+/-) served as a positive control for both reactions, the non-template control as a negative control.

Three different genotypes were possible:

- Wild-type (+/+).
  Showed only a positive band in the bottom part (e.g. pup #2).

- Nogo knock-out (-/-).
  Showed only a positive band in the upper part (e.g. pup #3).

- Heterozygous Nogo knock-out (+/-).
  Showed a positive band in the upper and lower part (e.g. pup #1).

For the SC/DRGN co-cultures, Schwann cells of WT pups were used as a control and compared to cells from either Nogo KO or heterozygous Nogo KO pups from the same litter.

Problems with DNA extraction
In the first few months of experimental work, the main problem was that the DNA bands on the electrophoresis gel showed a weak signal intensity. Sometimes it was not clear whether there is a positive DNA band or just contamination. As a consequence, genotyping had to be performed two or three times to be absolutely clear.

Different approaches of DNA isolation (Section 6.2.1) concerning temperature and time during DNA dissolution were tried (e.g. dissolution at 4°C for two days or at RT o/n), but the problem had to do with isopropanol induced DNA precipitation, as we found out. The Eppendorf tube containing a mixture of tail biopsy lysate and isopropanol was shaken too vigorously. As a result, the precipitated

DNA thread ruptured into small pieces. After recovering the remaining DNA thread from the solution and dissolving it, the yield of DNA extracted from the tail biopsies was too low to give a strong PCR signal on the electrophoresis gel.

When slowly tilting the tube instead of vigorously shaking it, visibly more DNA precipitated and solid DNA bands were obtained on the electrophoresis gel.

7.1.2 Schwann cell culture

Littermate pups (postnatal (p)3 or p4) were used to isolate Schwann cells from the sciatic nerves and culture them o/n (Section 6.3.2). For each genotype (either WT and Nogo KO or WT and heterozygous Nogo KO) a separate Schwann cell culture was established. To make sure that the final read-outs (total neurite length, longest branch and total number of intersections) are comparable, the isolated cells were counted and plated at the same density for both genotypes.

Cell density played a critical role
The density of the plated Schwann cells was a critical point, because if the density was too high, some Schwann cells aggregated and formed clumps (Figure 7.3).

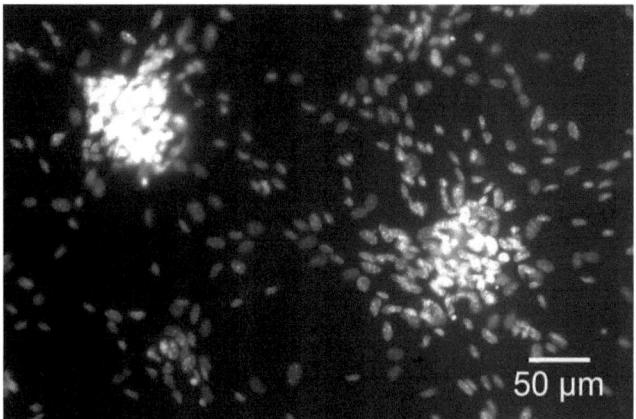

Figure 7.3: Aggregation of Schwann cells. Cells are visualized through nuclear Hoechst staining.

Neurons grown on such aggregates showed an increased branching phenotype (Figure 7.4c,d). To prevent this phenomenon, Schwann cells were cultured at a density of $1.2 \cdot 10^5$ cells/cm^2. Cultures established at such densities resulted in a homogeneous Schwann cell layer (Figure 7.4a) and typically lacked aggregates.

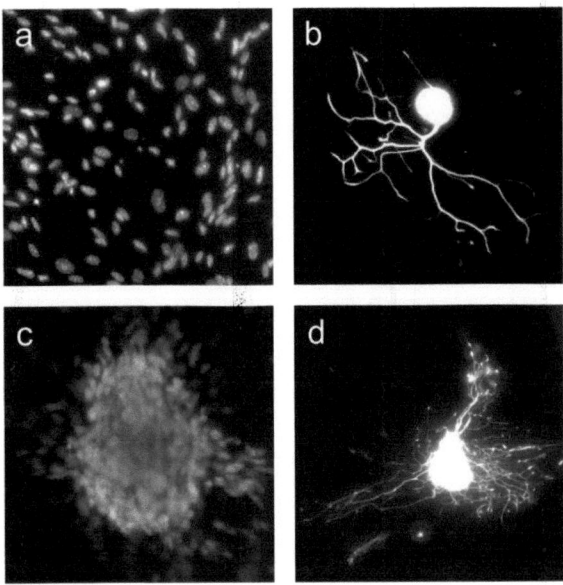

Figure 7.4: Branching behavior of neurons was affected by the morphology of the underlying Schwann cell layer. (**a**) Homogeneous layer of Schwann cells. (**b**) Neuron that grew on a homogeneous Schwann cell layer. (**c**) Aggregation of Schwann cells. (**d**) Neuron that grew on aggregated Schwann cells. The images a and c are visualized through nuclear Hoechst staining, b and d through N52 staining.

7.1.3 SC/DRGN co-culture

After incubation of Schwann cells for either 1 day(s) in vitro (div) (referred to as "Short-time co-culture") or 4 div (referred to as "Long-time co-culture"), sensory neurons were isolated from the DRG of an adult wild-type mouse (between two and three months old, see Section 6.3.3 for the sensory neuron isolation protocol) and added to the Schwann cell cultures.

Depending on the experimental set-up, the neurons were added either with physical (referred to as "Direct co-culture", see Section 6.3.3.1) or without physical contact (referred to as "Indirect co-culture", see Section 6.3.3.2) to the Schwann cells. Figure 7.5 illustrates the differences between these two experimental set-ups in schematic front views.

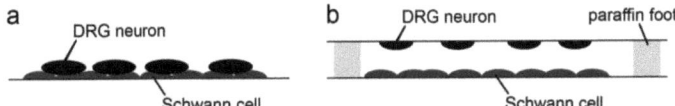

Figure 7.5: Differences between experimental set-ups. (**a**) Front view of a direct co-culture. (**b**) Front view of an indirect co-culture. Schwann cells are shown in blue, DRGN in black.

7.1.4 Immunostaining

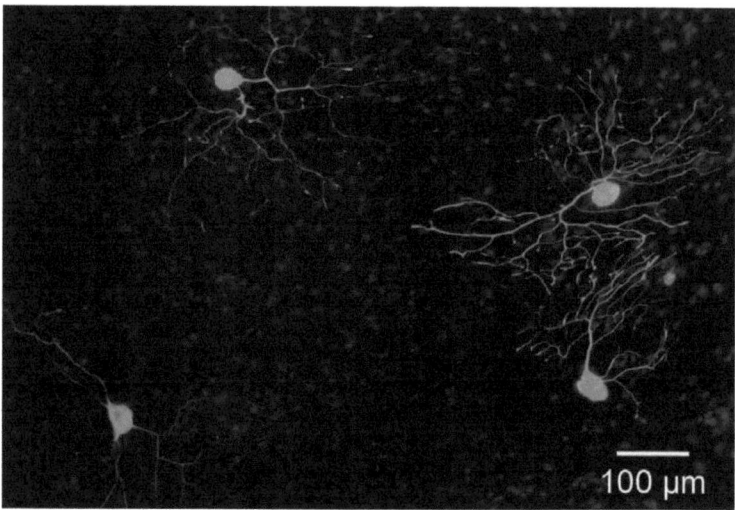

Figure 7.6: SC/DRGN direct co-culture at 10x magnification. Neurons are stained with N52 (green), cell nuclei with Hoechst (blue).

Different primary antibodies were used for experiments of the direct and the indirect co-culture set-up (Section 6.4.3). Indirect co-culture experiments were stained with N52 and TuJ-1, whereas direct co-culture experiments were stained only with N52 antibody (Figure 7.6).

TuJ-1 also stained Schwann cells
TuJ-1 could not be used in the direct experimental set-up, because it turned out to be not specific for neurons. The TuJ-1 antibody also bound to Schwann cells, which led to problems with immunofluorescence microscopy, because the neurons could not be clearly distinguished from the underlying Schwann cells (Figure 7.7).

Due to the different experimental set-ups (Figure 7.5), staining with TuJ-1 was not a problem for indirect co-culture experiments, because there were no Schwann cells on the coverslips.

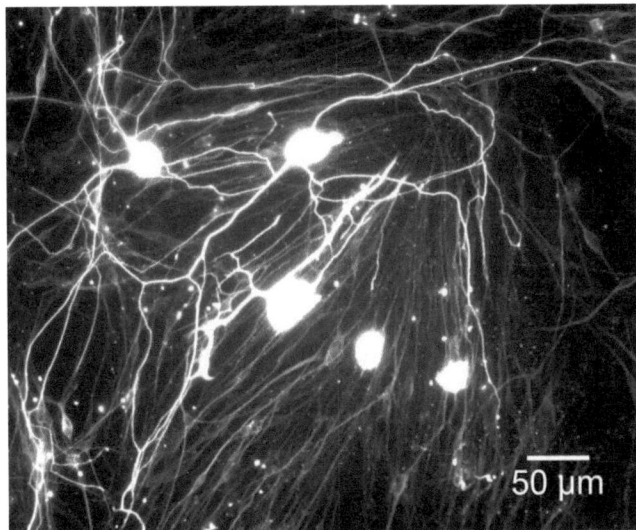

Figure 7.7: Problems with TuJ-1 antibody. TuJ-1 prominently stains DRGN, but also gives a marked signal for Schwann cells.

7.1.5 Neuron analysis

Images of the fluorescent-labeled neurons from the co-cultures were taken and analyzed using Sholl analysis (Section 6.5).

Criteria for including neurons in the analysis

Only neurons which met the following criteria were used for analysis:

- Growth on a homogeneous layer of Schwann cells.
  Some Schwann cells aggregated and formed clumps. Neurons grown on such aggregates showed much more branching than neurons grown on a homogeneous Schwann cell layer and were excluded from analysis (see Figure 7.4).

- No compromised growth pattern.
  Neurons that grew near the edges of the coverslip showed a compromised growth pattern and were excluded from analysis (see Figure 7.8a).

- All neurites of a neuron had to be intact.
  Some neurites got damaged by the handling of the coverslip during procedures like fixation or mounting of co-cultures and were excluded from analysis (see Figure 7.8b).

- No overlapping of neurites from different neurons.
  Some neurons grew so close to each other that they could not be segregated to individual neurons. Both neurons were excluded from analysis (see Figure 7.8c).

- The longest neurite of the neuron had to be longer than the diameter of the cell body of that neuron. Neurons with shorter neurites were excluded from analysis (see Figure 7.8d).

- Strong staining signal of all neurites.
  The peripheral neurites of some neurons showed a weak staining signal, which made it difficult to distinguish them from the background noise. Such neurons are prone to neuritic artifacts in the skeletonization process (Section 6.5.2) and were consequently excluded from analysis (see Figure 7.8e).

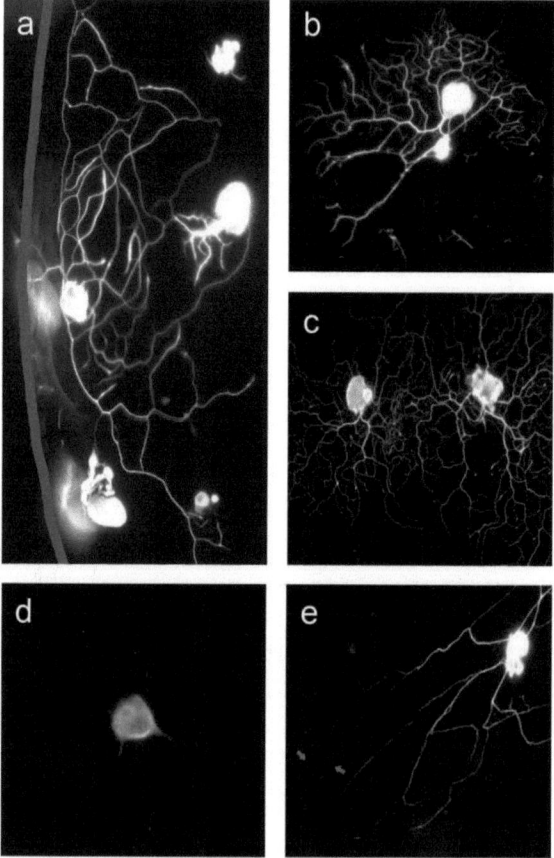

Figure 7.8: Type of neurons which did not meet the criteria for analysis. (**a**) Compromised growth pattern by the edge of the coverslip (shown in red). (**b**) Neuron with damaged neurites. (**c**) Overlapping neurites from different neurons. (**d**) The longest neurite was shorter than the diameter of the cell body. (**e**) Weak staining signal of peripheral neurites (indicated by red arrows).

7.2 Knock-out of Schwann cell expressed Nogo resulted in a reduced branching index of co-cultured sensory neurons

7.2.1 Short-time co-culture revealed a robust branching phenotype

To find out how the knock-out of Nogo in Schwann cells affects the morphology of neurons, direct short-time co-cultures of DRGN and WT or Nogo KO Schwann cells were established (see Section 7.1.3 for more information about the experimental set-up).

In total, five experiments were conducted and, as shown in Figure 7.9, the TNL (WT: 1.00, KO: 0.69 ± 0.07; $p = 0.012$) and the TNIS (WT: 1.00, KO: 0.71 ± 0.07; $p = 0.012$) were significantly decreased in DRGN cultured on Nogo KO Schwann cells. In contrast, no statistically significant difference regarding the LB (WT: 1.00, KO: 0.95 ± 0.05; $p = 0.379$) was seen between DRGN cultured on either WT or Nogo KO Schwann cells.

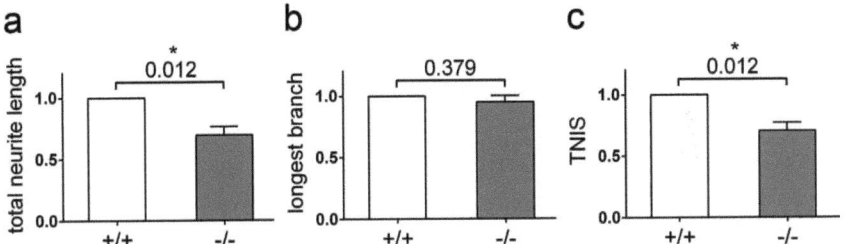

Figure 7.9: Morphological characteristics of DRGN cultured on either WT ($+/+$) or Nogo KO ($-/-$) Schwann cells (Direct short-time co-culture). Bar charts of (a) total neurite length, (b) longest branch and (c) total number of intersections are shown. Data represent mean $\pm$ SEM, KO is expressed relative to WT (WT is set to 1.0), $n = 5$, * is $p \leq 0.05$.

In all experiments conducted for this diploma thesis, the TNIS (number of neurite intersections with all concentric circles drawn around a neuron) instead of the number of neurite intersections for each concentric circle was compared between neurons cultured on different genotypes.

Figure 7.10 exemplarily shows the differences when comparing the number of neurite intersections for each concentric circle between neurons cultured on either WT or Nogo KO Schwann cells. Cultured DRGN from a single experiment (direct short-time co-culture) were used as a source for the diagram. In this experiment the number of neurite intersections of the circles with a radius of 40-90 μm, 110 μm, 140 μm and 160 μm were significantly lower in neurons cultured on Nogo KO Schwann cells as to compared to the wild-type littermate. Other experiments conducted with this experimental set-up yielded similar diagrams. However, this form of data representation was not chosen due to inter-experimental differences in the long distance growth pattern of neurons.

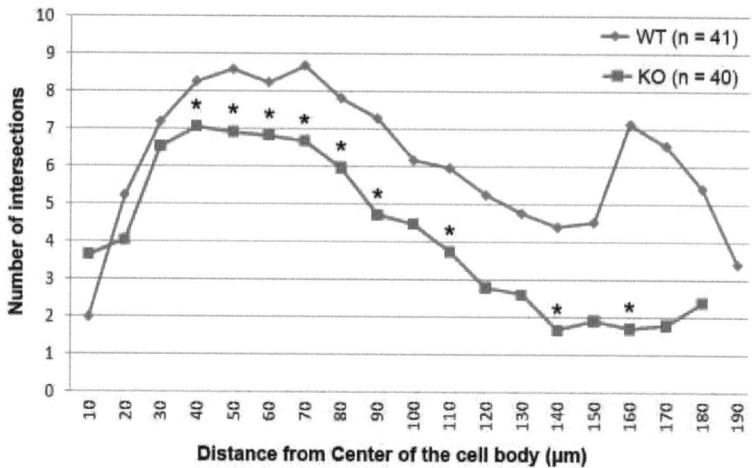

Figure 7.10: Detailed morphology of DRGN from a direct short-time co-culture. The diagram depicts the number of neurite intersections for each concentric circle drawn around the center of the neuronal cell body (see Figure 6.7). Means for neurons cultured on WT (blue line) or Nogo KO Schwann cells (red line) are shown. * is p ≤ 0.05, two-tailed two-sample t-test.

Another morphological characteristic of sensory neurons that was measured was the diameter of the cell body. As Figure 7.11 shows, the diameters of neuronal cell bodies were normally distributed in each co-culture. Most cell bodies lied in a range between 20 and 40 μm and no significant intra-experimental or inter-experimental differences were seen between neurons cultured on WT and Nogo KO Schwann cells.

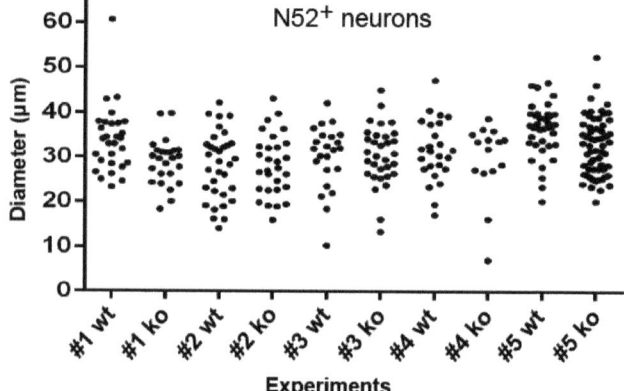

Figure 7.11: Distribution of cell body diameters of DRGN from direct short-time co-cultures. Single experiments are separated by the genotype (e.g. #1 wt and #1 ko). Every dot represents one cell body. Neurons were stained with N52 antibody.

7.2.2 The branching phenotype disappeared in a long-time co-culture

The decreased branching phenotype of DRGN cultured on Nogo KO Schwann cells that was seen in direct short-time co-culture experiments disappeared, when the Schwann cells were cultured for 4 days before the DRGN were added (Direct long-time co-culture).

As Figure 7.12 shows, no statistically significant difference of the TNL (WT: 1.00, KO: 1.04 ± 0.14; p = 0.814), the LB (WT: 1.00, KO: 1.00 ± 0.05; p = 0.96) or the TNIS (WT: 1.00, KO: 1.03 ± 0.14; p = 0.818) was found between neurons cultured on either WT or Nogo KO Schwann cells. In total, five experiments were conducted with this experimental set-up.

As in the direct short-time co-culture experiments, the diameters of neuronal cell bodies were normally distributed in each co-culture. Most cell bodies lied in a range between 20 μm and 40 μm and showed no statistically significant intra- or inter-experimental differences between neurons cultured on WT and Nogo KO Schwann cells (data not shown).

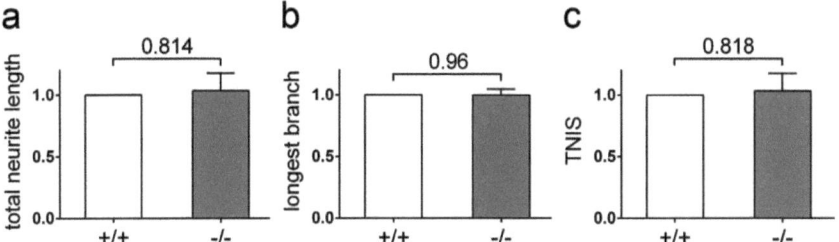

Figure 7.12: Morphological characteristics of DRGN cultured on either WT (+/+) or Nogo KO (-/-) Schwann cells (Direct long-time co-culture). Bar charts of (a) total neurite length, (b) longest branch and (c) total number of intersections are shown. Data represent mean ± SEM, KO is expressed relative to WT (WT is set to 1.0), n = 5.

7.3 Culturing DRGN on heterozygous Nogo KO Schwann cells showed no effect

When DRGN were cultured on heterozygous Nogo KO (+/-) Schwann cells, no statistically significant difference of the TNL (WT: 1.00, heterozygous KO: 0.92 ± 0.16; p = 0.67), the LB (WT: 1.00, heterozygous KO: 1.05 ± 0.06; p = 0.524) or the TNIS (WT: 1.00, heterozygous KO: 0.93 ± 0.16; p = 0.727) was seen compared to neurons grown on WT Schwann cells. The cultures were established as direct short-time co-cultures and in total four experiments were conducted.

The diameters of neuronal cell bodies were normally distributed in each co-culture. Most cell bodies lied in a range between 20 μm and 40 μm and showed no statistically significant intra- or inter-experimental differences between neurons cultured on WT and Nogo KO Schwann cells (data not shown).

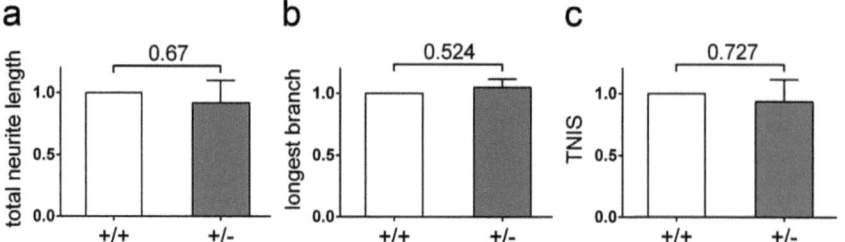

Figure 7.13: Morphological characteristics of DRGN cultured on either WT (+/+) or heterozygous Nogo KO (+/-) Schwann cells (Direct short-time co-culture). Bar charts of (a) total neurite length, (b) longest branch and (c) total number of intersections are shown. Data represent mean ± SEM, heterozygous Nogo KO is expressed relative to WT (WT is set to 1.0), n = 4.

7.4 Indirect experimental set-up revealed a different phenotype

Indirect short-time co-cultures were established (see Section 7.1.3 for more information about the experimental set-up) to find out whether the effect of decreased axonal branching of DRGN cultured on Nogo KO Schwann cells that was seen in direct short-time co-culture experiments (Section 7.2.1) is mediated by a direct, physical interaction between Schwann cells and neurons or via an indirect interaction by molecules secreted from Schwann cells.

Five experiments were conducted and as Figure 7.14 shows, the LB (WT: 1.00, KO: 1.18 ± 0.05; p = 0.03) was significantly increased in DRGN cultured on Nogo KO Schwann cells. The other two morphological characteristics, TNL (WT: 1.00, KO: 1.24 ± 0.11; p = 0.097) and TNIS (WT: 1.00, KO: 1.27 ± 0.11; p = 0.065), were close to significance.

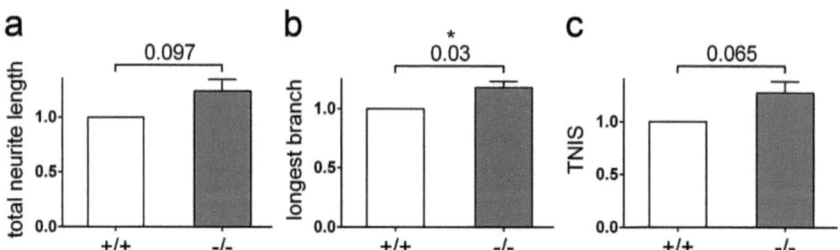

Figure 7.14: Morphological characteristics of DRGN cultured on either WT (+/+) or Nogo KO (-/-) Schwann cells (Indirect short-time co-culture). Bar charts of (a) total neurite length, (b) longest branch and (c) total number of intersections are shown. Data represent mean ± SEM, KO is expressed relative to WT (WT is set to 1.0), n = 5, * is p ≤ 0.05.

As Figure 7.15 shows, the diameters of neuronal cell bodies were normally distributed in each co-culture and showed no statistically significant intra- or inter-experimental differences. In contrast to all other experiments, where most of the cell bodies lied in a range between 20 μm and 40 μm, cell bodies of neurons from indirect short-time co-culture experiments lied in a wider range. In all experiments conducted with this experimental set-up, the cell bodies had diameters between 20 μm and 50 μm.

This observation is probably due to the different culture conditions. While neurons in the direct set-up were cultured on a layer of Schwann cells, they were grown on glass coverslips in the indirect approach. Furthermore, it is important to note that neurons from indirect co-culture experiments were stained with two antibodies (N52 and TuJ-1), whereas neurons from direct co-culture experiments were stained only with N52 (see Section 7.1.4 for more information).

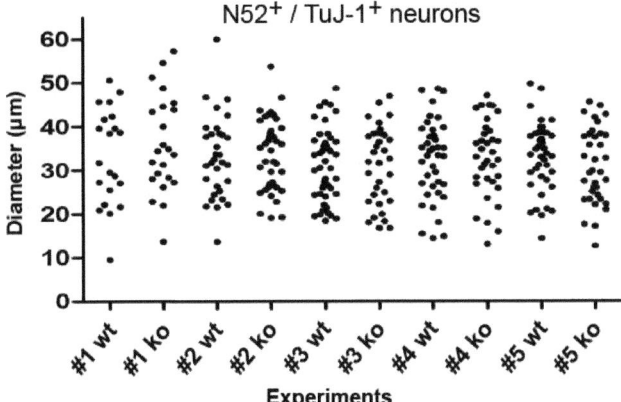

Figure 7.15: Distribution of cell body diameters of DRGN from indirect short-time co-cultures. Single experiments are separated by the genotype (e.g. #1 wt and #1 ko). Every dot represents one cell body. Neurons are stained with the antibodies N52 and TuJ-1.

8 Discussion

In the first part of the diploma thesis, direct short-time co-culture experiments of DRGN with either WT or Nogo KO Schwann cells identified Nogo as a promotor of axonal branching. It was shown that the TNIS and the TNL were significantly decreased in DRGN cultured on Nogo KO Schwann cells. These experiments also revealed that axon elongation is not affected by Nogo, since there was no difference of the LB between DRGN cultured on either WT or Nogo KO Schwann cells.

In contrast to the short-time experiments (SC were 1 div before DRGN were added), direct long-time experiments (SC were 4 div) showed no difference in any of the observed morphological parameters (TNL, LB and TNIS). We explain this observation by the down-regulation of Nogo protein expression in WT Schwann cells over time in culture, which is supported by immunocytochemistry experiments [Schweigreiter R, personal communication].

The second goal was to find out whether the branch-promoting effect of Nogo that was seen in direct short-time co-culture experiments is mediated by a direct, physical interaction between Schwann cells and neurons or via an indirect interaction by molecules secreted from Schwann cells.

To solve this question, we established indirect short-time co-culture experiments. These experiments revealed a different phenotype than what we had observed in the direct short-time co-culture experiments. The LB of DRGN cultured on Nogo KO Schwann cells was significantly increased. Additionally, the TNIS and the TNL showed a statistical trend towards significance ($p = 0.065$ and $p = 0.097$, respectively).

These results, however, are preliminary since the neuronal staining protocol was markedly different between the direct and the indirect approach. Specifically, neurons in the indirect approach were stained with both N52 and TuJ-1, whereas neurons in the direct approach were stained with N52 only. TuJ-1 was initially used as an additional antibody, because previous immunostainings showed a stronger signal intensity of peripheral neurites [Schweigreiter R, personal communication]. The reason that TuJ-1 could not be used in the direct experimental set-up was that it also stained Schwann cells, which led to difficulties with neuron analysis (see Section 7.1.4 for more information).

For a reliable comparison of data, neurons in the indirect set-up will thus have to be stained with N52 only, as was done with neurons in the direct approach.

The existence of different signaling pathways for axon branching and axon elongation provides an explanation how Nogo affects only axonal branching. The main signaling pathways for axon outgrowth during development and regeneration are the Ras/extracellular signal-regulated kinase (ERK) and the phosphatidylinositol-3 kinase (PI3K)/Akt pathway. The activation of the Ras/ERK pathway is associated with elongative axon growth, while the PI3K/Akt pathway is linked to axonal branching. Both pathways are activated by receptor tyrosine kinases (RTKs) upon binding of specific ligands. The PI3K/Akt pathway is primarily activated by plasma membrane-bound RTKs and the Ras/ERK pathway by endocytosis of activated RTKs into endosomes. Different studies showed that long-living signaling endosomes with sustained Ras/ERK pathway activation are required for axon elongation [1]. The decision whether axonal branching or long-distance growth of axons is affected depends on the balance of activation of these two pathways. Activation of the PI3K/Akt pathway over the Ras/ERK pathway, for example, favors axonal branching [1].

The fact that plasma membrane-bound RTKs primarily activate the PI3K/Akt pathway and affect axonal branching matches the finding that Nogo mediates its branch-promoting effect via a direct cell surface interaction between Schwann cells and neurons.

The branch-promoting effect of Nogo is possibly mediated by the activation of neuronal plasma membrane-bound receptor proteins. A characterization of plasma membrane proteins of WT and Nogo KO Schwann cells might reveal differences in the localization and/or activation of receptor-type proteins.

Within the different experimental set-ups, the measured diameters of the neuronal cell bodies showed high reliability and were normally distributed in a range between 20 µm and 40 µm (direct co-culture experiments) and between 20 µm and 50 µm (indirect co-culture experiments). No significant intra-experimental or inter-experimental differences were seen and the distribution of N52-immunoreactive cell bodies was consistent with previously published measurements [12], [13]. Based on the measured diameters, a more detailed analysis of subpopulations (e.g. small-diameter Aδ and large-diameter Aβ cells) could be made in addition.

It is important to note that the measured diameters of the neuronal cell bodies can not be considered as absolute values, because the images of the fluorescent-labeled neurons were overexposed in order to visualize the most peripheral neurites. This overexposure of peripheral neurites led to an expansion of the intensely stained cell bodies.

An open point remains the relative contribution of the two Nogo isoforms Nogo-A and Nogo-B to the observed branching phenotype. While Nogo-B is abundantly expressed in Schwann cells, we also found Nogo-A, albeit at lower levels [Schweigreiter R, unpublished]. Since we used a Nogo-A/B mutant mouse line [9], we can currently not distinguish between these two isoforms. To assess the influence of Nogo-A versus Nogo-B on the branching pattern, rescue experiments could be made. Specifically, Nogo-A/B KO Schwann cells in culture could be transfected with an adenoviral vector carrying the complementary DNA (cDNA) for Nogo-A or Nogo-B. In previous experiments we found that transfection of Schwann cells by green fluorescent protein (GFP)-expressing adenovirus is a good method for Schwann cell transfection [data not shown].

The means of the three morphological parameters (TNL, LB and TNIS) were not reported as absolute values. Results from WT data were set to 1.0 and the corresponding KO or heterozygous KO data was expressed as a relative value. This representation was chosen in order to normalize the inter-experimental differences of neuronal long-distance growth.

Although all experiments were performed under identical conditions, the maximum distance of neurite outgrowth varied from experiment to experiment. This was also the reason why the TNIS (number of neurite intersections with all concentric circles drawn around a neuron) instead of the number of neurite intersections for each concentric circle was compared between neurons cultured on different genotypes (see Section 7.2.1 and Figure 7.10 for more information).

The data presented in this thesis may eventually be of clinical relevance. As outlined in the introduction, reinnervation in the injured PNS is far from perfect and functional recovery is tedious and limited. A major problem of regenerating peripheral axons is the induction of excessive collateral sprouting by neurotrophic factors and neuropoietic cytokines, which are secreted by Schwann cells as part of the lesion response. While this cocktail of polypeptides generates a promotive environment for axonal distance growth, it stimulates at the same time axonal sprouting which results in misdirected reinnervation and impaired functional recovery. Ameliorating the sprouting effect without impeding the long-distance axonal elongation is thus a highly desirable goal for peripheral nerve lesion therapies. By blocking Schwann cell expressed Nogo we may have identified a mechanism that does just that. In contrast to the CNS, where Nogo is best known for inhibiting the long-distance growth of regenerating axons, Nogo in the PNS seems to specifically promote the branching of axonal fibers. Thus, blocking Nogo may be a therapeutic option for both the injured central and peripheral nervous system and the Nogo blocking strategies that have been conceived for the CNS may readily be applied to the peripheral scenario as well.

9 Bibliography

[1] Klimaschewski L, Hausott B, Angelov DN. The pros and cons of growth factors and cytokines in peripheral axon regeneration. Int Rev Neurobiol. 2013;108:137–171.

[2] Navarro X, Vivo M, Valero-Cabre A. Neural plasticity after peripheral nerve injury and regeneration. Prog Neurobiol. 2007;82:163–201.

[3] Chen ZL, Yu WM, Strickland S. Peripheral regeneration. Annu Rev Neurosci. 2007;30:209–233.

[4] Corfas G, Velardez MO, Ko CP, Ratner N, Peles E. Mechanisms and roles of axon-Schwann cell interactions. J Neurosci. 2004;24:9250–9260.

[5] Mirsky R, Jessen KR, Brennan A, Parkinson D, Dong Z, Meier C, et al. Schwann cells as regulators of nerve development. J Physiol Paris. 2002;96:17–24.

[6] Schweigreiter R. The natural history of the myelin-derived nerve growth inhibitor Nogo-A. Neuron Glia Biol. 2008;4:83–89.

[7] Huber AB, Weinmann O, Brosamle C, Oertle T, Schwab ME. Patterns of Nogo mRNA and protein expression in the developing and adult rat and after CNS lesions. J Neurosci. 2002;22:3553–3567.

[8] Acevedo L, Yu J, Erdjument-Bromage H, Miao RQ, Kim JE, Fulton D, et al. A new role for Nogo as a regulator of vascular remodeling. Nat Med. 2004;10:382–388.

[9] Zheng B, Ho C, Li S, Keirstead H, Steward O, Tessier-Lavigne M. Lack of enhanced spinal regeneration in Nogo-deficient mice. Neuron. 2003;38:213–224.

[10] M Galun RB, Brandt A. Multiscale edge detection and fiber enhancement using differences of oriented means. ICCV. 2007;.

[11] Rishal I, Golani O, Rajman M, Costa B, Ben-Yaakov K, Schoenmann Z, et al. WIS-NeuroMath enables versatile high throughput analyses of neuronal processes. Dev Neurobiol. 2013;73:247–256.

[12] Hammond DL, Ackerman L, Holdsworth R, Elzey B. Effects of spinal nerve ligation on immunohistochemically identified neurons in the L4 and L5 dorsal root ganglia of the rat. J Comp Neurol. 2004;475:575–589.

[13] Price TJ, Hargreaves KM, Cervero F. Protein expression and mRNA cellular distribution of the NKCC1 cotransporter in the dorsal root and trigeminal ganglia of the rat. Brain Res. 2006;1112:146–158.

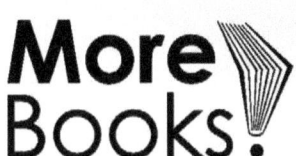
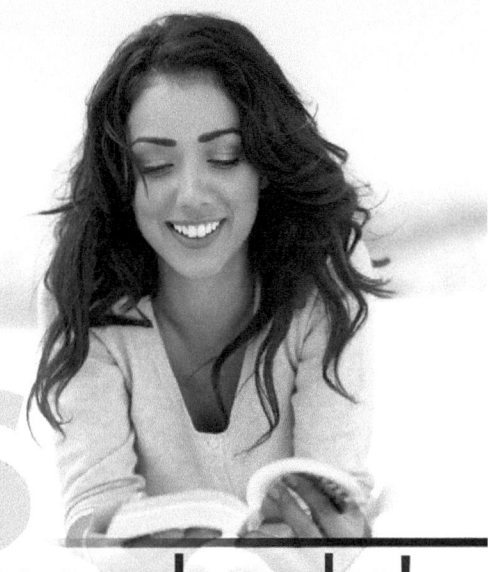
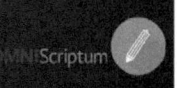

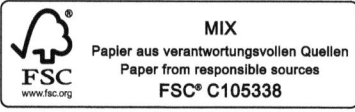
Printed by Books on Demand GmbH, Norderstedt / Germany